The PMDD Diet

Unlocking Relief and Well-Being through Nutrition and Lifestyle Choices

Emily Clark

Table of Contents

Introduction

Jenny's journey towards balancing hormones and mood through the PMDD Diet is a testament to her resilience and determination. For years, she had endured the overwhelming symptoms of Premenstrual Dysphoric Disorder (PMDD), which took a toll on her emotional well-being and daily life. But Jenny was determined to find a way to regain control and improve her quality of life.

Step 1: Education and Research

Jenny started her journey by educating herself about PMDD and the role of diet in managing hormonal imbalances and mood swings. She devoured books, articles, and research papers, seeking a deeper understanding of the condition and potential dietary solutions.

Step 2: Consulting a Healthcare Provider

With her newfound knowledge, Jenny took the next crucial step and consulted a healthcare provider who specialized in women's health. Together, they discussed her PMDD symptoms and created a personalized management plan that included dietary modifications.

Step 3: Embracing the PMDD Diet

Jenny fully embraced the PMDD Diet, making thoughtful choices about what she ate during different phases of her menstrual cycle. She learned to prioritize foods rich in essential nutrients like calcium, magnesium, B vitamins, and omega-3 fatty acids. These nutrients were known to play a role in hormonal regulation and mood stabilization.

Step 4: Mindful Eating

Jenny adopted mindful eating practices, paying close attention to how her body responded to different foods. She noticed that certain dietary choices had a profound impact on her energy levels, mood, and overall well-being during her menstrual cycle. This awareness allowed her to make more informed decisions about her diet.

Step 5: Tracking Progress

Jenny kept a detailed journal of her PMDD symptoms and dietary choices. This meticulous tracking helped her identify patterns and triggers. She noticed that her symptoms were less severe when she adhered to the PMDD Diet and avoided inflammatory foods like sugar and processed fats.

Step 6: Adding Supplements and Herbs

In collaboration with her healthcare provider, Jenny incorporated nutritional supplements and herbal remedies into her regimen. These supplements provided additional support in addressing hormonal imbalances and mood fluctuations. She closely followed her healthcare provider's recommendations and adjusted her supplement intake as needed.

Step 7: Lifestyle Changes

Understanding that diet was just one piece of the puzzle, Jenny made comprehensive lifestyle changes. She prioritized stress reduction through practices like meditation and yoga. Regular exercise became a part of her routine, and she ensured she got sufficient sleep to support hormonal balance.

Step 8: Seeking Support

Jenny recognized the importance of having a support system. She confided in close friends and family members about her PMDD journey, and they provided emotional support and encouragement. She also joined an online PMDD support group, connecting with others who shared similar experiences and insights.

As time passed, Jenny's dedication to the PMDD Diet and her holistic approach to wellness paid off. Her hormonal imbalances gradually stabilized, and her mood swings became less severe and manageable. While she still faced challenges during her menstrual cycle, they no longer controlled her life.

Jenny's story serves as an inspiration to anyone grappling with PMDD. It highlights the transformative power of education, dietary choices, supplements, and a holistic approach to wellness. Through her determination and a strong support system, Jenny found a way to balance her hormones and mood, ultimately regaining control over her life and experiencing improved well-being despite the challenges of PMDD. Her journey is a beacon of hope for others facing similar struggles, showing that with the right strategies, PMDD can be managed effectively, and a fulfilling life can be reclaimed.

Premenstrual Dysphoric Disorder (PMDD) is a condition that affects countless women around the world, yet its impact on daily life can be profoundly underestimated. If you're reading this guide, you or someone you care about may be dealing with the physical and emotional rollercoaster that PMDD can bring. But there's hope, and it starts with understanding the power of nutrition and lifestyle choices.

Understanding Premenstrual Dysphoric Disorder

PMDD is more than just "PMS on steroids." It's a complex and often debilitating condition characterized by severe mood disturbances, physical discomfort, and cognitive changes that typically occur in the days leading up to menstruation. These symptoms can disrupt every aspect of life, from relationships to work, and make each month feel like a battle.

The Role of Diet and Lifestyle in Managing PMDD

The good news is that while PMDD is a challenging condition, it is not without solutions. One of the most promising approaches to managing PMDD is through dietary and lifestyle modifications. This guide is here to empower you with knowledge about how the foods you eat and the way you live can significantly impact PMDD symptoms.

Throughout this guide, we will delve into the hormonal imbalances that underlie PMDD, explore the nutrients your body needs for balance, provide practical meal plans and recipes, discuss supplements and herbal remedies, and offer strategies for reducing stress and improving overall well-being.

By the time you finish reading, you'll be armed with the information and tools necessary to take control of your PMDD symptoms and regain a sense of normalcy during your menstrual cycle. PMDD may be challenging, but with the right approach, it can be managed effectively, allowing you to enjoy life to the fullest.

Let's embark on this journey together towards a healthier, happier you.

Chapter 1
Understanding Premenstrual Dysphoric Disorder (PMDD)

PMDD is a severe form of premenstrual syndrome (PMS) that affects some individuals with menstrual cycles. It is characterized by intense emotional and physical symptoms that typically occur in the days leading up to menstruation. Unlike regular PMS, PMDD symptoms are so severe that they can significantly disrupt daily life and functioning.

Key Points to Understand about PMDD:

1. **Symptoms:** PMDD symptoms can include severe mood swings, irritability, anxiety, depression, fatigue, and physical discomfort like bloating and breast tenderness.

2. **Timing:** These symptoms usually start in the luteal phase of the menstrual cycle (after ovulation) and typically improve or disappear after the onset of menstruation.

3. **Severity:** PMDD is distinguished by the severity and impact of its symptoms. It's not simply feeling a bit

moody before your period; it's a condition that can be genuinely debilitating.

4. **Diagnosis:** PMDD can be diagnosed by a healthcare provider through a careful evaluation of symptoms and their timing in relation to the menstrual cycle. Keeping a symptom diary can aid in the diagnosis.

5. **Hormonal Imbalance:** While the exact cause of PMDD is not fully understood, hormonal fluctuations, especially in serotonin levels, are believed to play a significant role.

6. **Treatment:** Treatment options for PMDD may include lifestyle changes, dietary adjustments, stress management, medication, and therapy. The approach to treatment is often personalized to address an individual's specific symptoms and needs.

7. **Impact on Quality of Life:** PMDD can have a profound impact on a person's relationships, work, and overall well-being. Seeking support from healthcare professionals, friends, and family is essential for managing the condition effectively.

Understanding PMDD is the first step towards managing it effectively. If you or someone you know is experiencing severe premenstrual symptoms that significantly affect daily life, it's crucial to seek medical advice for proper diagnosis and treatment.

1.1 What Is PMDD?

PMDD, or Premenstrual Dysphoric Disorder, is a severe form of premenstrual syndrome (PMS) that affects some individuals in the days or weeks leading up to their menstrual period. It is characterized by a range of physical, emotional, and psychological symptoms that significantly disrupt daily life and functioning. PMDD is a diagnosable medical condition that goes beyond the more common and milder symptoms associated with PMS.

Key features of PMDD include:

1. **Emotional Symptoms:** PMDD can cause intense mood swings, irritability, anger, anxiety, and depression. These emotional symptoms often interfere with relationships and daily activities.

2. **Physical Symptoms:** Individuals with PMDD may experience physical discomfort such as breast

tenderness, bloating, headaches, and joint or muscle
pain.

3. **Cognitive Symptoms:** Cognitive changes can
occur, including difficulty concentrating, forgetfulness,
and confusion.

4. **Behavioral Symptoms:** Some people with PMDD
may engage in impulsive behaviors, experience a loss of
interest in activities they typically enjoy, or feel
overwhelmed by daily responsibilities.

5. **Timing of Symptoms:** PMDD symptoms
typically occur in the luteal phase of the menstrual cycle,
which is the two weeks before menstruation begins.
Symptoms usually improve or disappear once
menstruation starts.

6. **Severity and Duration:** To be diagnosed with
PMDD, the symptoms must be severe enough to
significantly interfere with daily life, and they must
occur consistently in the menstrual cycle for at least two
consecutive months.

The exact cause of PMDD is not fully understood, but it
is believed to be related to hormonal fluctuations,
particularly in estrogen and progesterone levels, during
the menstrual cycle. These hormonal changes can affect

brain chemistry, leading to mood disturbances and other symptoms.

PMDD is a medical condition that requires evaluation and diagnosis by a healthcare provider. Treatment options may include lifestyle changes, dietary modifications, medication, therapy, and, in some cases, hormonal treatments. It's essential for individuals experiencing severe PMS symptoms to seek medical attention to determine if they have PMDD and to explore appropriate management strategies to improve their quality of life.

-Defining PMDD and its distinction from PMS
- Prevalence and who is affected by PMDD
- Common PMDD symptoms and their severity

1.2 The Impact of PMDD on Daily Life

The impact of PMDD (Premenstrual Dysphoric Disorder) on daily life can be profound and challenging. PMDD is a severe form of premenstrual syndrome (PMS) characterized by a range of physical, emotional, and cognitive symptoms. These symptoms typically occur in the two weeks leading up to menstruation and can significantly disrupt a person's daily routine and overall well-being. Here are some ways in which PMDD can affect daily life:

1. **Emotional Turmoil:** PMDD often brings intense mood swings, irritability, and emotional instability. A person with PMDD may experience severe depression, anxiety, and anger. These emotional fluctuations can strain relationships and make it difficult to engage in social activities.

2. **Cognitive Impairments:** PMDD can lead to cognitive difficulties, including trouble concentrating, forgetfulness, and mental fogginess. This can impact work or academic performance and make it challenging to complete tasks that require focus and attention.

3. **Physical Discomfort:** Physical symptoms of PMDD, such as breast tenderness, bloating, headaches, and joint or muscle pain, can be debilitating. The pain and discomfort may limit physical activities and make it hard to engage in regular exercise or even perform simple daily tasks.

4. **Impact on Work and Productivity:** The emotional and cognitive symptoms of PMDD can affect a person's ability to work effectively. Reduced productivity, missed days at work or school, and difficulties with decision-making may be common during PMDD episodes.

5. **Social Relationships:** The irritability, mood swings, and emotional distress associated with PMDD can strain personal relationships. Loved ones may find it challenging to understand or cope with the sudden and intense changes in mood and behavior.

6. **Quality of Life:** PMDD can significantly reduce an individual's overall quality of life. The cyclical nature of the disorder means that affected individuals experience periods of relative well-being followed by episodes of distress, making it challenging to maintain a consistent and fulfilling life.

7. **Isolation:** Some individuals with PMDD may withdraw from social activities and isolate themselves during symptomatic periods to cope with their emotional and physical discomfort. This can further impact their social and emotional well-being.

8. **Treatment Seeking:** Managing PMDD often involves seeking medical help, which can be time-consuming and emotionally taxing. Finding effective treatments and coping mechanisms may require a significant amount of effort and persistence.

It's important to note that the severity and specific symptoms of PMDD can vary among individuals. While some may experience all of these challenges, others may have milder symptoms that are more manageable.

Seeking professional help, such as consulting a healthcare provider or mental health expert, is crucial for individuals with PMDD. Treatment options, including lifestyle changes, dietary modifications, medication, therapy, and hormonal treatments, can help alleviate symptoms and improve overall daily functioning and well-being.

- Personal stories and testimonials to illustrate the real-life impact
- How PMDD affects relationships, work, and overall quality of life

1.3 The Hormonal Connection

The hormonal connection is a key factor in understanding PMDD (Premenstrual Dysphoric Disorder). PMDD is a condition characterized by severe mood, physical, and cognitive symptoms that occur in the luteal phase of the menstrual cycle, typically in the two weeks leading up to menstruation. The hormonal changes that take place during this phase are believed to be a central driver of PMDD symptoms. Here's how the hormonal connection plays a crucial role in PMDD:

1. **Estrogen and Progesterone Fluctuations:** Throughout the menstrual cycle, the levels of the hormones estrogen and progesterone rise and fall. It's during the luteal phase, particularly in the days leading up to menstruation, that these hormonal fluctuations become more pronounced.

2. **Impact on Brain Chemistry:** The changes in estrogen and progesterone levels are thought to influence brain chemistry. Specifically, they can affect neurotransmitters like serotonin, which play a vital role in mood regulation. Lower serotonin levels are associated with symptoms of depression and irritability, both of which are common in PMDD.

3. **Emotional and Mood Symptoms:** The hormonal fluctuations can trigger emotional and mood disturbances in individuals with PMDD. These can include intense mood swings, irritability, anxiety, and feelings of sadness or hopelessness. The severity of these symptoms can make it challenging to manage daily life effectively.

4. **Physical Symptoms:** Hormonal changes can also contribute to physical symptoms associated with PMDD,

such as breast tenderness, bloating, and headaches. These symptoms can add to the overall discomfort and distress experienced during the luteal phase.

5. **Cognitive Changes:** Some individuals with PMDD experience cognitive changes, including difficulties with concentration, forgetfulness, and mental fog. These cognitive impairments can affect work, academic performance, and daily tasks that require focus and attention.

6. **Response to Hormonal Treatments:** The hormonal connection is further evident in the fact that some individuals with PMDD respond positively to treatments that regulate hormone levels. Hormonal treatments, such as birth control pills or hormone replacement therapy, aim to stabilize hormonal fluctuations and can help alleviate PMDD symptoms in some cases.

It's important to note that while hormonal fluctuations are a central feature of PMDD, other factors, such as genetics and individual sensitivities, may also contribute to the condition. The exact mechanisms behind PMDD are still being studied, but the hormonal connection remains a focal point in understanding and managing this complex disorder.

Managing PMDD often involves addressing the hormonal component through dietary modifications, supplements, or hormonal treatments, in addition to lifestyle changes and emotional support. It is essential for individuals experiencing severe PMDD symptoms to seek medical attention and work with healthcare providers to find the most effective treatment approach for their unique needs.
- Overview of the menstrual cycle and hormone fluctuations
- The role of hormones in triggering PMDD symptoms
- Research and studies on hormonal imbalances in PMDD

1.4 Diagnosis and Differential Diagnosis

Diagnosis and differential diagnosis are critical aspects of identifying and distinguishing PMDD (Premenstrual Dysphoric Disorder) from other conditions with similar symptoms. Proper diagnosis is essential for effective management and treatment. Here's an overview of both:

Diagnosis of PMDD:

1. **Clinical Assessment:** The process begins with a clinical assessment by a healthcare provider. The provider will gather a detailed medical history, including

the patient's menstrual cycle patterns and the nature, severity, and timing of their symptoms.

2. **Diagnostic Criteria:** PMDD is diagnosed based on specific diagnostic criteria outlined in the Diagnostic and Statistical Manual of Mental Disorders (DSM-5). To meet the criteria, a patient must experience at least five out of 11 defined emotional and physical symptoms during the luteal phase of their menstrual cycle. These symptoms must be severe enough to significantly disrupt daily life and functioning.

3. **Symptom Tracking:** Keeping a symptom diary or chart is often recommended. This helps establish a pattern of recurring symptoms across several menstrual cycles and can aid in the diagnosis.

4. **Exclusion of Other Conditions:** Healthcare providers will also perform a differential diagnosis to rule out other conditions that may have similar symptoms, such as depression, anxiety disorders, bipolar disorder, or other mood disorders.

5. **Medical Examination:** A medical examination may be conducted to rule out underlying medical conditions that could be contributing to the symptoms. This may include blood tests to assess hormone levels or to check for thyroid dysfunction.

6. **Psychological Assessment:** In some cases, a psychological assessment or evaluation may be recommended to evaluate mood and emotional symptoms in more detail.

Differential Diagnosis:

Differential diagnosis is the process of distinguishing PMDD from other conditions that share similar symptoms. This is crucial because effective treatment strategies can differ based on the underlying condition. Conditions that may be considered in the differential diagnosis of PMDD include:

1. **Major Depressive Disorder:** Depression shares some symptoms with PMDD, such as mood swings, irritability, and fatigue. However, the timing of symptoms (primarily occurring in the luteal phase) is a key differentiator.

2. **Generalized Anxiety Disorder:** Anxiety disorders can have symptoms like tension, nervousness, and irritability, which may overlap with PMDD. Again, the timing of symptoms is a distinguishing factor.

3. **Bipolar Disorder:** Bipolar disorder may involve mood swings, but the pattern of symptoms and their duration can differ from PMDD.

4. **Other Mood Disorders:** Various mood disorders, such as cyclothymic disorder or borderline personality disorder, may have symptoms that overlap with PMDD and need to be considered.

5. **Other Medical Conditions:** Conditions like thyroid disorders or chronic pain conditions can lead to mood changes and fatigue, which may resemble PMDD symptoms.

The differential diagnosis process requires a careful evaluation by a healthcare provider who considers the timing, severity, and specific nature of symptoms, as well as medical history and any potential coexisting conditions. Accurate diagnosis is essential to ensure that individuals receive the appropriate treatment and support for their specific condition.

- How PMDD is diagnosed by healthcare professionals
- Distinguishing PMDD from other mood disorders and conditions
- The importance of accurate diagnosis for effective management

1.5 The Psychological Aspect of PMDD

The psychological aspect of PMDD (Premenstrual Dysphoric Disorder) plays a significant role in understanding this condition. PMDD is not only characterized by physical symptoms but also by a range of emotional and psychological symptoms that can profoundly affect a person's mental well-being. Here's a closer look at the psychological aspect of PMDD:

1. **Mood Disturbances:** PMDD often leads to severe mood disturbances. During the luteal phase of the menstrual cycle, individuals with PMDD may experience intense mood swings, irritability, and emotional volatility. These mood changes can be rapid and severe, making it challenging to regulate emotions and maintain stable relationships.

2. **Depression:** Depressive symptoms are common in PMDD. Individuals may experience feelings of sadness, hopelessness, and worthlessness during this phase of their cycle. These symptoms can mimic those of major depressive disorder but are specific to the luteal phase.

3. **Anxiety:** Anxiety symptoms are also prevalent in PMDD. People with PMDD may feel anxious, nervous,

or on edge. This can manifest as excessive worrying, restlessness, or even panic attacks.

4. **Emotional Sensitivity:** Individuals with PMDD may become highly emotionally sensitive during symptomatic periods. Everyday stressors and challenges can feel overwhelming, and even minor issues may provoke intense emotional reactions.

5. **Anger and Irritability:** PMDD can lead to episodes of intense anger and irritability. These emotional outbursts can strain personal and professional relationships and often occur without apparent provocation.

6. **Cognitive Impairments:** Some individuals with PMDD experience cognitive changes, including difficulties with concentration, memory, and decision-making. These cognitive impairments can interfere with work, school, and daily tasks.

7. **Social Withdrawal:** Because of the emotional and psychological distress associated with PMDD, some individuals may withdraw from social activities and isolate themselves during symptomatic periods. This isolation can further exacerbate feelings of loneliness and depression.

8. **Impact on Relationships:** The psychological symptoms of PMDD can take a toll on personal relationships. Loved ones may find it challenging to understand or cope with the intense mood swings, anger, and emotional distress experienced by someone with PMDD.

It's important to note that the psychological symptoms of PMDD are cyclical, typically occurring in the days or weeks leading up to menstruation and subsiding once menstruation begins. This cyclical pattern distinguishes PMDD from other mood disorders, such as major depressive disorder or generalized anxiety disorder.

Effective management of the psychological aspect of PMDD often involves a combination of approaches, including lifestyle changes, dietary modifications, psychological therapy, and, in some cases, medication. Seeking support from healthcare providers and mental health professionals is crucial for individuals with PMDD to develop strategies for coping with these challenging psychological symptoms and improving their overall quality of life.
- Discussing the emotional and cognitive symptoms of PMDD
- How PMDD can impact mental health and well-being
- Coping strategies for dealing with PMDD-related emotional challenges

1.6 The Physical Aspect of PMDD

The physical aspect of PMDD (Premenstrual Dysphoric Disorder) is characterized by a range of physical symptoms that occur in the days or weeks leading up to menstruation. These symptoms can be uncomfortable and distressing, and they contribute to the overall burden of PMDD. Here's an overview of the physical aspect of PMDD:

1. **Breast Tenderness:** Many individuals with PMDD experience breast tenderness and swelling. This physical symptom can be painful and uncomfortable, making it difficult to engage in regular activities and wear certain types of clothing.

2. **Bloating:** Bloating is a common physical symptom of PMDD. It can lead to a feeling of fullness and abdominal discomfort. Some people with PMDD may notice a visible increase in abdominal size due to bloating.

3. **Headaches:** Headaches, including tension headaches and migraines, are reported by some individuals with PMDD. These headaches can be severe and contribute to overall discomfort.

4. **Joint and Muscle Pain:** PMDD can cause joint and muscle pain. This physical discomfort can affect mobility and make it challenging to engage in physical activities or exercise.

5. **Fatigue:** Fatigue is a common physical symptom of PMDD. Individuals may feel excessively tired and lack energy during the days leading up to menstruation. This fatigue can interfere with daily responsibilities.

6. **Gastrointestinal Symptoms:** Some people with PMDD experience gastrointestinal symptoms such as diarrhea or constipation. These symptoms can further contribute to discomfort and distress.

7. **Appetite Changes:** PMDD may lead to changes in appetite, including food cravings or loss of appetite. These changes can affect dietary choices and overall nutritional intake.

8. **Sleep Disturbances:** Sleep disturbances, including insomnia or disrupted sleep patterns, can occur during the luteal phase of the menstrual cycle in individuals with PMDD. This can lead to increased fatigue and mood disturbances.

It's important to note that the severity and specific physical symptoms of PMDD can vary among individuals. While some may experience all of these physical symptoms, others may have a subset of them, and their intensity can vary from one menstrual cycle to another.

Managing the physical aspect of PMDD often involves a combination of strategies, including lifestyle changes, dietary modifications, pain relief measures, and in some cases, medication. Engaging in regular exercise, maintaining a balanced diet, and practicing stress reduction techniques can also help alleviate physical symptoms and improve overall well-being during the symptomatic phase. Seeking guidance from a healthcare provider is essential to develop a personalized management plan that addresses the individual's specific physical symptoms and needs.

- Exploring the physical symptoms of PMDD, such as bloating and pain
- How physical symptoms can exacerbate emotional distress
- Lifestyle changes and dietary considerations for managing physical symptoms

Chapter 2
Hormonal Imbalances and PMDD

Premenstrual Dysphoric Disorder (PMDD) is strongly associated with hormonal imbalances in the body. While the exact cause of PMDD is not fully understood, it is believed to be linked to fluctuations in hormones, particularly estrogen and progesterone, during the menstrual cycle.

Key Points to Understand:

1. **Estrogen and Progesterone:** Hormones like estrogen and progesterone play crucial roles in regulating various bodily functions, including mood and emotions. Fluctuations in these hormones can impact brain chemistry, leading to mood disturbances.

2. **Serotonin Levels:** One prevailing theory suggests that PMDD may be related to changes in serotonin, a neurotransmitter that affects mood. Hormonal

fluctuations can influence serotonin levels, potentially leading to mood swings and emotional symptoms.

3. **Hormonal Trigger:** PMDD symptoms typically emerge during the luteal phase of the menstrual cycle, which occurs after ovulation and is characterized by increased progesterone levels. It is during this phase that individuals with PMDD may experience heightened emotional and physical symptoms.

4. **Hormonal Treatments:** Hormonal treatments, such as hormonal birth control and medications that regulate hormone levels, are sometimes used to manage PMDD. These treatments aim to stabilize hormonal fluctuations and alleviate symptoms.

5. **Individual Variability:** It's important to note that not everyone with hormonal fluctuations will develop PMDD. Individual differences in sensitivity to hormonal changes and genetic factors may also play a role in who is more susceptible to PMDD.

Understanding the connection between hormonal imbalances and PMDD is crucial for developing effective management strategies. By addressing these imbalances through lifestyle changes, dietary adjustments, and, in some cases, medical treatments, individuals with PMDD can work towards reducing the severity of their symptoms and improving their overall quality of life.

2.1 The Menstrual Cycle and Hormone Fluctuations

Understanding the menstrual cycle and hormone fluctuations is crucial when discussing PMDD (Premenstrual Dysphoric Disorder) because these hormonal changes play a central role in the development of PMDD symptoms. Here's an overview of the menstrual cycle and how hormone fluctuations contribute to PMDD:

The Menstrual Cycle:

The menstrual cycle is a monthly series of physiological changes that occur in a woman's body in preparation for possible pregnancy. It typically lasts about 28 days, although variations are common. The cycle is divided into several phases:

1. **Menstruation (Day 1-5):** The cycle begins with menstruation when the uterine lining is shed. This phase is characterized by the shedding of the endometrial tissue and the release of blood from the uterus.

2. **Follicular Phase (Day 1-13):** Following menstruation, the body enters the follicular phase. During this phase, the brain's pituitary gland releases follicle-stimulating hormone (FSH), which stimulates the ovaries to produce several follicles, each containing an immature egg.

3. **Ovulation (Day 14):** Around the middle of the cycle, typically on day 14, a surge in luteinizing hormone (LH) triggers the release of a mature egg from one of the ovarian follicles. This is known as ovulation and is a crucial event in the menstrual cycle.

4. **Luteal Phase (Day 15-28):** After ovulation, the body enters the luteal phase. During this phase, the ruptured follicle transforms into a structure called the corpus luteum, which releases progesterone and some estrogen. These hormones prepare the uterine lining for possible pregnancy. If pregnancy does not occur, hormone levels drop, leading to the shedding of the uterine lining and the start of a new menstrual cycle.

Hormone Fluctuations and PMDD:

In PMDD, hormone fluctuations during the luteal phase are believed to be a significant factor in the development of symptoms. Specifically:

1. **Estrogen and Progesterone:** Both estrogen and progesterone levels rise and fall during the menstrual cycle. In PMDD, it is thought that some individuals may be more sensitive to these hormonal fluctuations. The drop in estrogen and progesterone levels during the late luteal phase is associated with PMDD symptoms.

2. **Impact on Brain Chemistry:** These hormonal changes can influence brain chemistry, particularly serotonin levels. Serotonin is a neurotransmitter that plays a crucial role in regulating mood. Decreased serotonin levels are associated with mood disturbances, including depression and irritability, which are common in PMDD.

3. **Symptom Onset:** PMDD symptoms typically appear in the late luteal phase of the menstrual cycle, a week or two before menstruation. They often subside shortly after menstruation begins, aligning with the hormonal fluctuations in the body.

Understanding these hormonal fluctuations is essential for healthcare providers when diagnosing and managing PMDD. Treatment strategies may aim to stabilize hormone levels or address the specific symptoms that arise during the luteal phase to provide relief and improve overall quality of life for individuals with PMDD.

- A detailed explanation of the phases of the menstrual cycle
- The role of estrogen, progesterone, and other hormones
- How hormone levels fluctuate throughout the menstrual cycle

2.2 The Hormonal Imbalance Hypothesis

The hormonal imbalance hypothesis is a leading theory that seeks to explain the underlying cause of PMDD (Premenstrual Dysphoric Disorder). This hypothesis suggests that PMDD is primarily triggered by fluctuations in hormonal levels, particularly estrogen and progesterone, during the menstrual cycle. Here's a closer look at the hormonal imbalance hypothesis:

Key Points of the Hormonal Imbalance Hypothesis:

1. **Sensitivity to Hormonal Changes:** According to this hypothesis, individuals with PMDD may be more sensitive or responsive to the natural hormonal fluctuations that occur during the menstrual cycle. While many individuals experience some mood and physical changes in response to these hormones, those with PMDD are believed to have heightened reactivity to the hormonal changes.

2. **Role of Estrogen and Progesterone:** Estrogen and progesterone are two key hormones that fluctuate throughout the menstrual cycle. It is thought that the interactions between these hormones, specifically the drop in their levels during the late luteal phase of the cycle (the two weeks before menstruation), contribute to the development of PMDD symptoms.

3. **Impact on Brain Chemistry:** The hormonal fluctuations, particularly the drop in estrogen and progesterone, are believed to influence brain chemistry, including neurotransmitter systems such as serotonin. Serotonin is associated with mood regulation, and changes in its levels can lead to mood disturbances, such as depression and irritability, which are common in PMDD.

4. **Cyclical Nature of Symptoms:** The hormonal imbalance hypothesis aligns with the cyclical nature of PMDD symptoms. Symptoms typically appear during the late luteal phase and subside shortly after menstruation begins, reflecting the hormonal changes in the body.

Supporting Evidence:

Several pieces of evidence support the hormonal imbalance hypothesis:

- Hormonal treatments, such as oral contraceptives or hormone replacement therapy, can be effective in alleviating PMDD symptoms by stabilizing hormonal levels.
- Some individuals with PMDD experience symptom improvement during pregnancy when hormonal levels remain relatively stable.
- Studies have shown that women with PMDD have differences in hormonal sensitivity and altered responses to hormonal challenges compared to those without PMDD.

Limitations and Ongoing Research:

While the hormonal imbalance hypothesis is a leading theory, it's essential to recognize that PMDD is a complex condition, and multiple factors may contribute to its development. Not all individuals with PMDD show consistent hormonal imbalances, and other factors, such as genetics, neurotransmitter function, and stress, may also play roles.

Ongoing research continues to explore the precise mechanisms behind PMDD and why some individuals are more sensitive to hormonal fluctuations than others. This research aims to improve our understanding of the condition and develop more targeted and effective treatments for PMDD.

- Exploring the theory that hormonal imbalances contribute to PMDD
- Research and studies supporting the hormonal imbalance hypothesis
- Understanding serotonin's role and its connection to mood changes

2.3 Identifying Triggers in the Menstrual Cycle

Identifying triggers in the menstrual cycle is a crucial step in understanding and managing PMDD (Premenstrual Dysphoric Disorder). PMDD is characterized by severe emotional, physical, and cognitive symptoms that typically occur during the luteal phase of the menstrual cycle, which is the two weeks before menstruation starts. Identifying triggers can help individuals anticipate and manage their symptoms more effectively. Here are some common triggers to watch for:

1. **Hormonal Fluctuations:** Hormonal changes are the primary triggers for PMDD. Pay attention to the timing of your symptoms in relation to your menstrual cycle. Symptoms often start after ovulation and intensify as you approach menstruation.

2. **Stress:** High levels of stress can exacerbate PMDD symptoms. Keep track of stressful events or periods of increased stress in your life and how they correlate with the severity of your symptoms.

3. **Dietary Choices:** Certain foods and dietary habits can influence PMDD symptoms. Some individuals may be more sensitive to caffeine, sugar, and processed foods. Keep a food diary to identify potential dietary triggers.

4. **Sleep Patterns:** Irregular sleep patterns or insufficient sleep can worsen PMDD symptoms. Monitor your sleep quality and duration to see if it affects the severity of your symptoms.

5. **Exercise and Physical Activity:** Regular physical activity can help alleviate PMDD symptoms, but excessive or strenuous exercise during the luteal phase may worsen symptoms in some individuals. Find a balance that works for you.

6. **Alcohol and Substance Use:** Alcohol and certain substances can disrupt hormone balance and affect mood. Be aware of how alcohol or substance use may impact your symptoms.

7. **Medications:** Some medications, including hormonal contraceptives and antidepressants, can influence PMDD symptoms. Discuss any changes in your medication regimen with your healthcare provider.

8. **Psychological Factors:** Emotional stressors, unresolved past traumas, or psychological conditions can interact with PMDD symptoms. Consider how your emotional well-being and psychological factors may contribute to your symptoms.

9. **Environmental Factors:** Exposure to environmental toxins or endocrine-disrupting chemicals can affect hormone regulation. Be mindful of your surroundings and potential sources of exposure.

10. **Lifestyle Changes:** Major life events or changes in routine can impact PMDD symptoms. Keep track of any significant life changes and how they coincide with symptom severity.

11. **Social Support:** The level of social support you have can influence your ability to cope with PMDD symptoms. Maintain a support network and consider how it affects your overall well-being.

To identify triggers, it's essential to maintain a symptom diary or calendar that tracks your symptoms throughout your menstrual cycle. Documenting when symptoms start, their severity, and any potential triggers can help you and your healthcare provider develop a personalized management plan. Understanding your specific triggers empowers you to make informed lifestyle adjustments, seek appropriate treatments, and improve your quality of life despite PMDD.

- Discussing how PMDD symptoms align with hormonal changes
- Recognizing the window of vulnerability for symptom onset
- The importance of tracking and predicting PMDD episodes

2.4 Other Factors That May Influence Hormones and PMDD

While hormonal fluctuations play a central role in PMDD (Premenstrual Dysphoric Disorder), there are several other factors that can influence hormones and contribute to the development or exacerbation of PMDD symptoms. Understanding these additional factors is important for a comprehensive perspective on PMDD and its management. Here are some of the key factors:

1. **Genetics:** Genetics can play a significant role in a person's susceptibility to PMDD. There may be a genetic

component that makes some individuals more prone to experiencing severe symptoms in response to hormonal fluctuations.

2. **Neurotransmitter Function:** The functioning of neurotransmitters in the brain, particularly serotonin, can impact mood regulation and may interact with hormonal changes to exacerbate PMDD symptoms. Serotonin levels can be influenced by factors like stress, dietary choices, and genetic variations.

3. **Stress:** High levels of stress can affect hormone balance and exacerbate PMDD symptoms. Chronic stress can lead to hormonal disturbances and disrupt the delicate interplay between hormones in the menstrual cycle.

4. **Diet and Nutrition:** Dietary choices can influence hormone levels and overall well-being. Poor nutrition, including high sugar and caffeine intake, may exacerbate PMDD symptoms, while a balanced diet rich in nutrients can support hormone balance.

5. **Environmental Toxins:** Exposure to certain environmental toxins, such as endocrine-disrupting chemicals found in some plastics and pesticides, may interfere with hormone regulation and contribute to PMDD symptoms.

6. **Sleep Disruptions:** Irregular sleep patterns and insufficient sleep can affect hormone production and regulation, potentially worsening PMDD symptoms.

7. **Physical Health Conditions:** Certain underlying medical conditions, such as thyroid disorders or polycystic ovary syndrome (PCOS), can disrupt hormone balance and contribute to PMDD-like symptoms.

8. **Medications:** Some medications, including hormonal contraceptives and antidepressants, can impact hormonal levels and potentially affect PMDD symptoms. In some cases, medications can be prescribed to manage PMDD.

9. **Lifestyle Factors:** Smoking and excessive alcohol consumption can affect hormone metabolism and increase the severity of PMDD symptoms.

10. **Psychological Factors:** Psychological factors, such as past trauma or emotional stressors, can influence the experience of PMDD symptoms. Addressing underlying psychological issues may be an important part of managing PMDD.

It's essential to recognize that PMDD is a multifaceted condition with a range of contributing factors. While hormonal fluctuations are a central component, addressing the broader context, including genetics, lifestyle, and psychological factors, can be crucial in understanding and managing PMDD effectively. A comprehensive approach to treatment often involves addressing these multiple factors through lifestyle changes, therapy, medication, and other interventions tailored to the individual's specific needs.

- Factors such as stress, genetics, and lifestyle choices
- How these factors can exacerbate hormonal imbalances
- Strategies for addressing these influences

2.5 The Role of Hormonal Treatments

Hormonal treatments play a significant role in managing PMDD (Premenstrual Dysphoric Disorder). These treatments are designed to regulate hormone levels, primarily estrogen and progesterone, to help alleviate the symptoms and improve the quality of life for individuals with PMDD. Here's an overview of the role of hormonal treatments in PMDD management:

1. **Oral Contraceptives (Birth Control Pills):** Birth control pills are a commonly prescribed hormonal treatment for PMDD. They work by stabilizing hormone

levels throughout the menstrual cycle. Typically, combination birth control pills containing both estrogen and progestin are used. Continuous or extended-cycle birth control regimens that reduce the number of menstrual periods per year may be particularly beneficial in managing PMDD.

2. **Progestin-Only Contraceptives:** Progestin-only contraceptives, such as the progestin-only pill (mini-pill), intrauterine devices (IUDs), or contraceptive implants, can be used to regulate hormones and reduce PMDD symptoms. These methods are often recommended when estrogen-containing contraceptives are not suitable for the individual.

3. **Hormone Replacement Therapy (HRT):** In some cases, hormone replacement therapy may be considered for women approaching menopause who also experience PMDD symptoms. HRT can help stabilize hormonal fluctuations associated with perimenopause.

4. **Gonadotropin-Releasing Hormone (GnRH) Agonists:** GnRH agonists are medications that temporarily suppress ovarian function and hormonal fluctuations. They can be effective in reducing PMDD symptoms, but they are usually used for short periods due to potential side effects like bone density loss.

5. **Selective Estrogen Receptor Modulators (SERMs):** SERMs, such as tamoxifen, can be used to regulate estrogen levels. These medications are more commonly used in breast cancer treatment but may be considered for PMDD when other treatments are ineffective.

6. **Dosing and Duration:** The specific dosing and duration of hormonal treatments will vary depending on the individual's needs and the severity of their PMDD symptoms. Treatment plans should be developed in consultation with a healthcare provider who specializes in women's health.

It's important to note that while hormonal treatments can be highly effective in managing PMDD, they are not suitable for everyone. The choice of treatment depends on various factors, including the individual's overall health, medical history, and preferences. Additionally, hormonal treatments may have potential side effects and risks, which should be discussed with a healthcare provider.

Hormonal treatments should be part of a comprehensive approach to PMDD management. Lifestyle modifications, dietary changes, stress reduction techniques, and psychotherapy can also play essential roles in managing PMDD symptoms and improving overall well-being. Individualized treatment plans should be developed based on a thorough evaluation by a healthcare provider to address the specific needs and goals of each person with PMDD.

- An overview of hormonal treatments for PMDD
- Discussing birth control options and hormone-regulating medications
- Benefits, risks, and considerations for each treatment approach

Chapter 3
Building a PMDD-Friendly Diet

Building a PMDD-Friendly Diet
A PMDD-friendly diet is one that focuses on incorporating specific nutrients and foods while avoiding or limiting others to help alleviate the symptoms of

Premenstrual Dysphoric Disorder (PMDD). While dietary changes alone may not completely cure PMDD, they can significantly reduce the severity of symptoms and improve overall well-being during the menstrual cycle.

Key Points to Understand:

1. **Nutritional Impact:** The foods we eat can impact hormone levels, inflammation, and neurotransmitter activity, all of which are linked to PMDD symptoms. A PMDD-friendly diet aims to address these factors through smart dietary choices.

2. **Balanced Nutrition:** A well-balanced diet rich in essential vitamins, minerals, and antioxidants is fundamental for supporting hormonal balance and mood stability.

3. **Key Nutrients:** Certain nutrients, such as calcium, magnesium, B vitamins, and omega-3 fatty acids, have been shown to help reduce PMDD symptoms. These nutrients are often found in foods like leafy greens, fatty fish, whole grains, and nuts.

4. **Inflammatory Foods:** Some foods, like those high in refined sugars and processed fats, can trigger inflammation, exacerbating PMDD symptoms. Avoiding

or limiting these inflammatory foods is an essential aspect of a PMDD-friendly diet.

5. **Hydration:** Staying adequately hydrated is crucial for overall health and can help alleviate symptoms like bloating and mood swings associated with PMDD.

A PMDD-friendly diet is part of a holistic approach to managing PMDD symptoms, alongside other lifestyle changes, stress management, and, in some cases, medical treatments. It empowers individuals to take control of their nutrition, supporting hormonal balance and improving their quality of life during their menstrual cycle.

3.1 The Impact of Nutrition on PMDD

- Exploring the link between diet and PMDD symptoms
- How certain nutrients can affect hormonal balance and mood
- The role of inflammation and dietary choices in PMDD

3.2 Nutrients to Nourish Hormonal Balance

- Key vitamins and minerals that play a role in hormonal health

- Foods rich in these nutrients and their benefits
- How to incorporate these foods into your diet

3.3 Foods to Include for PMDD Relief

- A detailed list of PMDD-friendly foods
- Sample meal plans and recipes that prioritize these foods
- The importance of a balanced and diverse diet

3.4 Foods to Avoid or Limit

- Identifying foods that can exacerbate PMDD symptoms
- Understanding the impact of caffeine, alcohol, and sugar
- Strategies for reducing or eliminating trigger foods

3.5 The Role of Hydration

- The connection between hydration and PMDD symptoms
- Tips for staying adequately hydrated and its impact on overall well-being

Chapter 4
Meal Planning for PMDD Relief

Meal Planning for PMDD Relief
Meal planning for PMDD relief involves creating structured and thoughtfully designed meal plans that prioritize foods and nutrients known to alleviate the symptoms of Premenstrual Dysphoric Disorder (PMDD). This approach aims to support hormonal balance, reduce inflammation, and stabilize mood during the menstrual cycle.

Key Points to Understand:

1. **Structured Planning:** Meal planning involves organizing your daily and weekly meals in advance, ensuring that you include a variety of PMDD-friendly foods.

2. **Balanced Nutrition:** A well-rounded meal plan incorporates a mix of essential nutrients, including calcium, magnesium, B vitamins, and omega-3 fatty acids, which have been linked to PMDD symptom relief.

3. **Consistency:** Consistently following a PMDD-friendly meal plan throughout the menstrual cycle can help maintain hormonal stability and reduce symptom severity.

4. **Sample Meal Plans:** Sample meal plans offer a clear outline of what to eat at different times of the day, making it easier to stick to a PMDD-friendly diet.

5. **Mindful Eating:** Practicing mindful eating techniques can help prevent overeating or emotional eating, which may exacerbate PMDD symptoms.

6. **Meal Prep:** Preparing PMDD-friendly meals in advance can save time and reduce stress during symptomatic periods.

7. **Customization:** Meal plans should be customizable to accommodate individual dietary preferences, restrictions, and needs.

A well-structured meal plan for PMDD relief is an essential tool for individuals looking to manage their symptoms through dietary choices. It empowers individuals to proactively address the hormonal and nutritional aspects of PMDD and can significantly improve their quality of life during the menstrual cycle.

4.1 The Importance of Meal Planning

- Exploring the benefits of structured meal planning for PMDD management
- How meal planning can help ensure a balanced and PMDD-friendly diet
- The role of consistency in reducing symptoms

4.2 Sample PMDD-Friendly Meal Plans

- Providing sample meal plans for different stages of the menstrual cycle
- Breakfast, lunch, dinner, and snack ideas that prioritize PMDD-friendly foods
- Customizable options for individual preferences and dietary restrictions

4.3 Recipes for PMDD-Friendly Meals

- A collection of recipes designed to support hormonal balance and mood stability
- Step-by-step instructions and ingredient lists for easy meal preparation
- Tips for incorporating PMDD-friendly ingredients into everyday cooking

4.4 Portion Control and Mindful Eating

- Discussing the importance of portion control for managing PMDD symptoms
- Strategies for practicing mindful eating to avoid overeating or emotional eating
- The connection between balanced meals and stable mood

4.5 Meal Prep and Convenience

- How meal prep can save time and reduce stress during PMDD episodes
- Tips for batch cooking and storing PMDD-friendly meals
- Identifying convenient, healthy options for busy days

Supplements and herbs are additional tools in the toolkit for managing the symptoms of Premenstrual Dysphoric

Disorder (PMDD). They are considered complementary approaches to dietary and lifestyle changes and may provide relief from PMDD symptoms when used thoughtfully and under professional guidance.

Key Points to Understand:

1. **Nutritional Supplements:** Certain vitamins and minerals, such as calcium, magnesium, B vitamins, and omega-3 fatty acids, have been associated with PMDD symptom relief. Supplements can help ensure that individuals meet their nutritional needs.

2. **Herbal Remedies:** Herbal remedies, derived from plants, have been used for centuries to alleviate various health issues, including PMDD. Some herbs, like chasteberry (Vitex agnus-castus) and evening primrose oil, are thought to have potential benefits in managing PMDD symptoms.

3. **Holistic Approach:** Supplements and herbs are often used in conjunction with dietary modifications and lifestyle changes to provide a comprehensive approach to PMDD management.

4. **Safety and Professional Guidance:** It's crucial to use supplements and herbs safely and consult with healthcare providers before incorporating them into your

PMDD management plan. Some supplements and herbs may have interactions or side effects, and individual responses can vary.

5. **Monitoring and Adjustments:** Regular monitoring of the effects of supplements and herbs is essential. Adjustments to dosages or types of supplements may be necessary based on individual responses and changing symptoms.

6. **Complementary Strategies:** Supplements and herbs can complement other PMDD management strategies, such as stress reduction techniques, exercise, and dietary changes, to provide holistic relief.

Supplements and herbs are not a one-size-fits-all solution for PMDD, but they offer potential benefits for those seeking additional support. Always consult with a healthcare professional before starting any new supplement or herbal regimen to ensure that it aligns with your individual needs and health status.

5.1 Nutritional Supplements for Hormonal Balance

- Exploring the role of supplements in supporting PMDD management
- Key vitamins and minerals to consider as supplements
- Dosage recommendations and safety precautions

5.2: Herbal Remedies for PMDD Relief

- Introduction to herbal remedies as a complementary approach
- Herbs known for their potential benefits in alleviating PMDD symptoms
- Guidance on sourcing and using herbal remedies safely

5.3 Complementary Approaches

- Combining nutritional supplements and herbal remedies for a holistic approach
- How supplements and herbs can work together to address hormonal imbalances
- Consultation with healthcare professionals for personalized recommendations

5.4 Potential Risks and Interactions

- Discussion of potential risks associated with supplements and herbs
- Identifying contraindications and interactions with other medications
- The importance of informed and cautious use

5.5 Monitoring and Adjusting

- Strategies for monitoring the effectiveness of
supplements and herbs
- Making adjustments to the supplement and herbal
regimen based on individual responses
- Seeking guidance from healthcare providers for
ongoing management

Chapter 6
Lifestyle Strategies for PMDD Management

Lifestyle strategies are a vital component of managing
the symptoms of Premenstrual Dysphoric Disorder
(PMDD). These strategies encompass various practices
and choices that can help individuals reduce symptom
severity, improve emotional well-being, and enhance
overall quality of life during the menstrual cycle.

Key Points to Understand:

1. **Stress Reduction Techniques:** Stress can exacerbate PMDD symptoms. Stress reduction techniques like mindfulness, meditation, deep breathing exercises, and relaxation practices can help manage stress levels and promote emotional stability.

2. **Exercise and PMDD:** Regular physical activity is known to have a positive impact on mood and hormonal balance. Engaging in exercises that suit individual preferences and fitness levels can be beneficial for PMDD management.

3. **Sleep and PMDD:** Quality sleep is essential for hormonal balance and overall well-being. Implementing good sleep hygiene practices and creating a sleep routine can help minimize fatigue and mood disturbances associated with PMDD.

4. **Hormone-Healthy Habits:** Lifestyle choices, such as avoiding smoking, limiting alcohol intake, and moderating caffeine consumption, can support hormonal balance and reduce potential PMDD triggers.

5. **Mind-Body Connection:** Practices like yoga, tai chi, and other mind-body exercises can promote physical and emotional balance. These techniques enhance

resilience and help individuals cope with PMDD-related challenges.

6. **Complementary to Dietary Approaches:** Lifestyle strategies complement dietary modifications and other treatments for a holistic approach to PMDD management. Integrating these practices into daily life can significantly improve symptom relief.

7. **Individualized Approach:** The effectiveness of lifestyle strategies may vary from person to person. It's important to tailor these practices to individual preferences and needs.

By implementing these lifestyle strategies, individuals with PMDD can create a supportive environment that helps them better navigate the challenges posed by the condition. These strategies empower individuals to actively participate in their PMDD management and improve their overall well-being.

6.1 Stress Reduction Techniques

- Exploring the link between stress and PMDD symptoms
- Strategies for managing stress through relaxation, mindfulness, and meditation
- Incorporating stress-reduction practices into daily life

6.2 Exercise and PMDD

- The role of regular physical activity in managing
PMDD symptoms
- Types of exercise that may be particularly beneficial
- Creating an exercise routine that aligns with your
PMDD management goals

6.3 Sleep and PMDD

- How sleep quality and quantity affect PMDD
symptoms
- Sleep hygiene tips for improving restorative sleep
- Establishing a sleep routine to minimize PMDD-related
fatigue

6.4: Hormone-Healthy Habits

- Lifestyle choices that support hormonal balance
- The impact of smoking, alcohol, and caffeine on
PMDD symptoms
- Strategies for reducing or eliminating these triggers
from your routine

6.5 Mind-Body Connection

- Exploring the mind-body connection and its relevance to PMDD management
- Practices like yoga and tai chi that promote balance and well-being
- Techniques for maintaining emotional resilience during PMDD episodes

Chapter 7
Tracking and Managing PMDD Symptoms

Tracking and managing PMDD symptoms is a crucial aspect of effectively coping with Premenstrual Dysphoric Disorder (PMDD). By monitoring symptoms, identifying triggers, seeking professional guidance when needed, and implementing self-care techniques, individuals with PMDD can take an active role in symptom management and improve their overall quality of life.

Key Points to Understand:

1. **Keeping a Symptom Diary:** Maintaining a symptom diary involves documenting PMDD symptoms, their severity, and their timing over several menstrual cycles. This helps individuals recognize patterns and better understand their condition.

2. **Identifying Triggers:** Tracking symptoms allows individuals to identify potential triggers, such as specific foods, stressors, or lifestyle factors. Once identified, these triggers can be avoided or managed to reduce symptom severity.

3. **Seeking Professional Guidance:** Consulting healthcare providers for an accurate diagnosis and treatment options is essential. Effective communication with healthcare professionals about PMDD symptoms and their impact is key to receiving appropriate care.

4. **Self-Care Techniques:** Implementing self-care practices, such as stress reduction, exercise, healthy eating, and relaxation techniques, can help alleviate PMDD symptoms and improve emotional well-being.

5. **Building a Support System:** Having a support network of friends, family, or support groups can provide emotional and practical assistance during challenging PMDD episodes. Open communication about PMDD with loved ones is beneficial.

By actively tracking symptoms, identifying triggers, collaborating with healthcare professionals, practicing self-care, and seeking support, individuals can enhance their ability to manage PMDD effectively. This chapter empowers readers with practical tools and strategies to take control of their PMDD symptoms and improve their overall quality of life.

7.1: Keeping a Symptom Diary

- The importance of tracking PMDD symptoms over several menstrual cycles
- How to create a symptom diary and what to include
- Recognizing patterns and triggers through consistent tracking

7.2: Identifying Triggers

- Exploring common triggers for PMDD symptoms
- How diet, stress, lifestyle, and hormonal fluctuations can influence symptom severity

- Strategies for avoiding or mitigating identified triggers

7.3 Seeking Professional Guidance

- The role of healthcare providers in PMDD management
- When to consult a healthcare professional for diagnosis and treatment options
- Effective communication with healthcare providers about PMDD symptoms and their impact

7.4 Self-Care Techniques

- Self-care practices to alleviate PMDD symptoms and improve well-being
- Creating a self-care routine that addresses physical and emotional needs
- The importance of self-compassion and self-nurturing during symptomatic periods

7.5 Building a Support System

- The significance of a support network in PMDD management
- How to communicate with friends and family about PMDD
- Joining support groups or seeking counseling for additional assistance

Chapter 8
Support and Resources

Support and resources are essential components of managing Premenstrual Dysphoric Disorder (PMDD). This chapter provides valuable information and guidance on accessing the help and knowledge needed to navigate PMDD effectively.

Key Points to Understand:

1. **Connecting with Support Groups:** Support groups and online communities offer a safe space for individuals with PMDD to share their experiences, gain insights, and receive emotional support from peers who understand their challenges.

2. **Professional Guidance:** Healthcare providers, including gynecologists, psychiatrists, and therapists, play a critical role in PMDD management. This section emphasizes the importance of seeking professional help, understanding treatment options, and advocating for individual needs.

3. **Additional Resources:** Readers are provided with a curated list of books, websites, apps, and other materials dedicated to PMDD. This comprehensive

resource guide helps individuals access reliable information and research about PMDD.

4. **Empowerment:** Empowering individuals to take an active role in their PMDD management is a central theme. The chapter offers encouragement, resilience-building tips, and a reminder to celebrate progress in the journey toward improved PMDD management.

By utilizing the support networks and resources presented in this chapter, individuals with PMDD can better understand their condition, access professional guidance, connect with peers, and take the necessary steps to effectively manage their symptoms and enhance their overall well-being.

8.1 Connecting with Support Groups

- The value of peer support in PMDD management
- How to find and join PMDD support groups and online communities
- Sharing experiences and gaining insights from others with PMDD

8.2 Professional Guidance

- The role of healthcare providers, including gynecologists, psychiatrists, and therapists, in PMDD management
- Understanding treatment options, including medication, therapy, and lifestyle recommendations
- How to prepare for medical appointments and advocate for your needs

8.3 Additional Resources

- A comprehensive list of books, websites, and apps dedicated to PMDD
- Finding reputable sources of information and research
- Accessing tools and materials to support PMDD management

8.4 Empowering Yourself to Manage PMDD

- Encouragement for taking an active role in your PMDD management
- Tips for building resilience and maintaining a positive outlook
- Recognizing progress and celebrating victories in the journey to better PMDD management

Chapter 9
Conclusion

In conclusion, the PMDD diet has emerged as a subject of interest in the pursuit of managing symptoms associated with premenstrual dysphoric disorder. While anecdotal evidence and some preliminary studies suggest that certain dietary changes may contribute to symptom relief, a comprehensive understanding of the topic requires careful consideration of the current state of research.

Several studies have explored the relationship between nutrition and PMDD, highlighting potential connections between dietary factors and symptom severity. Common recommendations include reducing caffeine intake, increasing the consumption of complex carbohydrates, and maintaining stable blood sugar levels. However, the overall body of evidence is still in its early stages, with limited large-scale, well-controlled trials.

Individual responses to dietary interventions can vary widely, and what works for one person may not be universally applicable. Moreover, the multifaceted nature of PMDD, which involves complex hormonal, neurotransmitter, and psychological factors, adds complexity to the issue.

It is crucial for individuals considering a PMDD diet to approach it with realistic expectations and in consultation with healthcare professionals. While dietary adjustments may complement conventional treatments, they should not replace evidence-based medical interventions. A holistic approach that includes lifestyle modifications, stress management, and, where necessary, medication, is likely to be the most effective strategy in addressing the diverse array of symptoms associated with PMDD.

In essence, the PMDD diet remains an evolving area of study within the broader context of women's health. As research continues, a more nuanced understanding of the interplay between diet and PMDD may emerge, providing clearer guidance for individuals seeking to manage their symptoms through dietary interventions.

www.ingramcontent.com/pod-product-compliance
Lightning Source LLC
Chambersburg PA
CBHW071054260726
48661CB00006B/2280